The Power of PEMF Therapy: Unlocking Your Body's Natural Healing Ability

Chapter 1: Understanding PEMF Therapy

What is PEMF Therapy?
Brief history of PEMF Therapy
How does PEMF Therapy work?
Types of PEMF devices
Differences between PEMF and other forms of therapy

Chapter 2: The Benefits of PEMF Therapy

Pain relief
Improved circulation
Reduced inflammation
Enhanced healing and recovery
Better sleep
Reduced stress and anxiety
Improved athletic performance
Enhanced cognitive function
Other potential benefits

Chapter 3: Safety and Side Effects of PEMF Therapy

Risks and side effects
Contraindications
Precautions and guidelines
Safety tips

Chapter 4: Using PEMF Therapy for Pain Management

How PEMF Therapy can help with pain
Types of pain that can be treated with PEMF Therapy
Research studies on PEMF Therapy and pain management

<u>CHAPTER 1: Understanding PEMF Therapy</u>

<u>What is PEMF Therapy?</u>

PEMF therapy stands for Pulsed Electromagnetic Field therapy. It is a non-invasive and drug-free therapy that uses low-frequency electromagnetic waves to stimulate the body's natural healing process. PEMF therapy has been used for decades in various forms of medical treatment, including pain management, tissue repair, and bone healing.

PEMF therapy works by producing electromagnetic waves that penetrate through the skin and into the body's tissues. These waves create a pulsating magnetic field that helps to stimulate the cells in the body, promoting cellular repair and regeneration. The therapy is designed to mimic the natural electromagnetic field that surrounds us, and this is believed to have a positive impact on the body's ability to heal itself.

PEMF therapy can be used to treat a wide range of health conditions, including chronic pain, arthritis, inflammation, sports injuries, and post-surgical recovery. The therapy is particularly effective for treating chronic pain, as it helps to reduce inflammation and promote healing in the affected tissues.

PEMF therapy can be administered using various devices, including mats, pads, and blankets that can be placed directly on the body. Some devices can be used for whole-body therapy, while others are designed for localized treatment. The therapy is typically administered in a series of sessions, with the duration and frequency of the treatment depending on the specific condition being treated.

PEMF therapy is generally considered safe and non-invasive, with few side effects reported. However, there are some precautions that should be taken when using the therapy, particularly for individuals with medical devices such as pacemakers or cochlear implants. It is important to consult with a healthcare professional before beginning any new medical treatment, including PEMF therapy.

Brief history of PEMF Therapy

PEMF therapy, which stands for Pulsed Electromagnetic Field therapy, has a long and fascinating history. While the technology is relatively new, the concept of using magnetic fields for healing purposes has been around for centuries.

The use of magnets for healing purposes can be traced back to the ancient Greeks, who used magnets to treat various ailments. It was believed that magnets had the power to attract and repel certain elements in the body, which could help to restore balance and promote healing.

The concept of using electromagnetic fields for healing purposes began to take shape in the 19th century, with the discovery of electromagnetic waves by James Clerk Maxwell. This led to a greater understanding of the relationship between electromagnetic fields and the human body, and the potential for using these fields for therapeutic purposes.

The first practical application of electromagnetic therapy came in the form of electroconvulsive therapy (ECT), which was developed in the 1930s as a treatment for mental illness. ECT involves passing an electric current through the brain to induce a seizure, and while it is still used today in certain cases, it is also associated with significant side effects.

It wasn't until the 1960s that the first true PEMF therapy device was developed. A researcher named Andrew Bassett discovered that low-frequency electromagnetic fields could stimulate bone healing, and he went on to develop a device that could be used for this purpose. This device, called the "Pulsed Electromagnetic Field System", was used primarily for bone healing and was not widely adopted outside of the medical community.

In the years that followed, more and more researchers began to explore the potential of PEMF therapy for a wider range of applications. In the 1980s, NASA began studying the effects of PEMF therapy on astronauts, who were experiencing bone loss and other health issues due to the zero-gravity environment of space. The research showed that PEMF therapy could be effective in preventing and even reversing bone loss, as well as improving circulation and reducing inflammation.

Today, PEMF therapy is used to treat a wide range of health conditions, including chronic pain, arthritis, depression, and sports injuries. The therapy is non-invasive and does not require drugs or surgery, making it an attractive option for many patients.

There are now a variety of PEMF therapy devices available, ranging from small portable devices that can be used at home, to larger devices used in clinics and hospitals. The technology continues to evolve, with new studies and applications being discovered all the time.

In conclusion, PEMF therapy has a long and fascinating history, with roots dating back to ancient times. While the technology is relatively new, the concept of using magnetic fields for healing purposes has been around for centuries. Today, PEMF therapy is used to treat a wide range of health conditions and is a safe and effective alternative to traditional medical treatments. As the technology continues to evolve, it is likely that we will discover even more ways to use PEMF therapy to improve our health and well-being.

PEMF Therapy, or Pulsed Electromagnetic Field Therapy, is a non-invasive and drug-free form of therapy that has been gaining popularity in recent years. It is a type of therapy that uses electromagnetic waves to stimulate and heal the body at a cellular level. In this essay, we will take a closer look at how PEMF Therapy works, the types of PEMF devices available, and the differences between PEMF Therapy and other forms of therapy.

How PEMF Therapy Works

At the core of PEMF Therapy is the concept of electromagnetic fields. Our bodies are made up of trillions of cells, each of which has an electrical charge. These charges are necessary for the cells to communicate with each other and carry out various functions in the body. When the body experiences injury, disease, or inflammation, these electrical charges become disrupted, leading to pain and discomfort.

PEMF Therapy works by using low-frequency electromagnetic waves to stimulate the body's cells and restore their natural electrical charges. These waves are delivered through specialized devices, which can be applied directly to the affected area of the body or used to treat the body as a whole.

When the electromagnetic waves are applied to the body, they create a pulsed magnetic field that penetrates the tissues and cells. This pulsed magnetic field stimulates the cells' natural processes, helping to increase blood flow, reduce inflammation, and promote healing. The electromagnetic waves can also help to increase the production of ATP (adenosine triphosphate), which is the energy currency of the body's cells.

<u>**Types of PEMF Devices**</u>

There are several types of PEMF devices available, each with its own unique features and benefits. Here are a few of the most common types of PEMF devices:

Mat Devices: Mat devices are designed to be placed on a bed or other flat surface and can be used to treat the entire body. These devices are often used for general wellness and relaxation.

Localized Devices: Localized devices are designed to be used on a specific area of the body, such as the neck, back, or knee. These devices are often used for pain relief and to promote healing in specific areas.

Portable Devices: Portable devices are designed to be used on the go and can be carried in a purse or backpack. These devices are often used for general wellness and relaxation.

High-Intensity Devices: High-intensity devices deliver a more powerful electromagnetic wave and can penetrate deeper into the tissues. These devices are often used for chronic pain and inflammation.

<u>**Differences between PEMF Therapy and other forms of therapy**</u>

PEMF Therapy is a unique form of therapy that offers several advantages over other forms of therapy. Here are a few of the main differences between PEMF Therapy and other forms of therapy:

Non-Invasive: PEMF Therapy is a non-invasive form of therapy that does not require any incisions or injections. This makes it a safer and less painful alternative to surgery or other invasive procedures.

Drug-Free: PEMF Therapy does not involve the use of drugs or medications. This means that there are no side effects or risks associated with using PEMF Therapy.

Effective for a Wide Range of Conditions: PEMF Therapy has been shown to be effective for a wide range of conditions, including chronic pain, inflammation, and anxiety. This makes it a versatile and effective form of therapy.

Easy to Use: PEMF Therapy devices are easy to use and can be used in the comfort of your own home. This makes it a convenient and accessible form of therapy.

In conclusion, PEMF Therapy is a safe, effective, and non-invasive form of therapy that uses electromagnetic waves to stimulate the body's cells and promote healing. With a variety of PEMF

CHAPTER 2: The benefits of PEMF therapy

PEMF Therapy, also known as Pulsed Electromagnetic Field Therapy, is a non-invasive and drug-free form of therapy that has been gaining popularity in recent years. This type of therapy uses low-frequency electromagnetic waves to stimulate the body's cells and promote healing. In this chapter, we will explore the many benefits of PEMF Therapy, including pain relief, improved circulation, reduced inflammation, enhanced healing and recovery, better sleep, reduced stress and anxiety, improved athletic performance, enhanced cognitive function, and other potential benefits.

Pain Relief

One of the most significant benefits of PEMF Therapy is pain relief. PEMF Therapy has been shown to be effective in reducing chronic pain, including arthritis, back pain, and joint pain. The electromagnetic waves stimulate the body's natural healing processes, increasing blood flow and reducing inflammation, leading to a reduction in pain.

Improved Circulation

PEMF Therapy has been shown to improve circulation in the body. The electromagnetic waves stimulate the production of nitric oxide, a molecule that helps to dilate blood vessels and increase blood flow. Improved circulation can help to deliver oxygen and nutrients to the body's cells, leading to improved overall health.

Reduced Inflammation

Inflammation is a natural response of the body to injury or infection. However, chronic inflammation can lead to a range of health problems, including heart disease, diabetes, and cancer. PEMF Therapy has been shown to be effective in reducing inflammation in the body, helping to reduce the risk of chronic health problems.

Enhanced Healing and Recovery

PEMF Therapy has been shown to enhance healing and recovery in the body. The electromagnetic waves stimulate the body's natural healing processes, increasing blood flow and promoting the production of new cells. This can help to speed up the healing process and reduce recovery time after an injury or surgery.

Better Sleep

PEMF Therapy has been shown to improve sleep quality and duration. The electromagnetic waves can help to regulate the body's natural sleep-wake cycle, leading to improved sleep patterns. This can be particularly beneficial for individuals who suffer from sleep disorders or have difficulty sleeping.

Reduced Stress and Anxiety

PEMF Therapy has been shown to reduce stress and anxiety in the body. The electromagnetic waves can help to regulate the body's natural stress response, leading to reduced stress and anxiety levels. This can be particularly beneficial for individuals who suffer from chronic stress or anxiety disorders.

Improved Athletic Performance

PEMF Therapy has been shown to improve athletic performance in individuals. The electromagnetic waves can help to improve circulation, reduce inflammation, and enhance recovery, leading to improved athletic performance. This can be particularly beneficial for athletes who are looking to improve their performance and reduce the risk of injury.

Enhanced Cognitive Function

PEMF Therapy has been shown to enhance cognitive function in individuals. The electromagnetic waves can help to improve blood flow to the brain, leading to improved cognitive function and memory. This can be particularly beneficial for individuals who are looking to improve their cognitive function and reduce the risk of cognitive decline.

Other Potential Benefits

PEMF Therapy has also been shown to have other potential benefits, including:
Improving immune function
Reducing the risk of osteoporosis
Improving skin health and reducing the signs of aging
Reducing the risk of depression
Reducing the risk of cancer

CHAPTER 3: Safety and side effects of PEMF therapy

Pulsed Electromagnetic Field (PEMF) Therapy is a non-invasive and safe form of therapy that uses low-frequency electromagnetic waves to stimulate the body's cells and promote healing. However, as with any medical treatment, there are certain risks and side effects associated with PEMF Therapy. In this chapter, we will explore the safety and side effects of PEMF Therapy, including risks and side effects, contraindications, precautions and guidelines, and safety tips.

Risks and Side Effects

PEMF Therapy is generally considered safe and is associated with few risks and side effects. However, some people may experience mild side effects, such as:

Tingling or prickling sensation
Muscle twitching
Fatigue
Headache
Nausea
These side effects are usually mild and temporary, and typically disappear shortly after the treatment. If you experience any side effects after a PEMF Therapy session, it is important to speak with your healthcare provider.

Contraindications

While PEMF Therapy is generally safe, there are certain contraindications, or conditions under which PEMF Therapy should not be used. These include:

Pregnancy
Pacemaker or other implanted electronic device
Epilepsy or history of seizures
Active cancer
Acute infections
Bleeding disorders
Organ transplant
If you have any of these conditions, it is important to speak with your healthcare provider before considering PEMF Therapy.

Precautions and Guidelines

There are several precautions and guidelines that should be followed when undergoing PEMF Therapy. These include:

Avoiding exposure to high-frequency electromagnetic fields, such as those from power lines and cell phones
Limiting exposure to electromagnetic fields from other medical devices
Drinking plenty of water before and after the treatment to aid in the elimination of toxins
Not using PEMF Therapy while operating heavy machinery or driving
Not using PEMF Therapy while under the influence of drugs or alcohol
It is also important to follow the guidelines provided by your healthcare provider regarding the frequency and duration of PEMF Therapy sessions.

<u>**Safety Tips**</u>

To ensure the safety of PEMF Therapy, there are several safety tips that should be followed. These include:

Using only PEMF devices that have been approved by regulatory agencies, such as the FDA
Following the manufacturer's instructions for use of the device
Not exceeding the recommended treatment time or intensity
Avoiding placing the device directly on the eyes or over any metal implants
Not using the device on infants or small children
It is important to consult with your healthcare provider before beginning PEMF Therapy and to follow their recommendations for the safe use of the therapy.

<u>**Conclusion**</u>

PEMF Therapy is a safe and non-invasive form of therapy that offers a range of benefits for individuals. However, as with any medical treatment, there are certain risks and side effects associated with PEMF Therapy. It is important to understand these risks and to follow the guidelines and safety tips provided by your healthcare provider to ensure the safe and effective use of PEMF Therapy. If you have any questions or concerns about the safety of PEMF Therapy, speak with your healthcare provider.

CHAPTER 4: Using PEMF therapy for pain management

Pulsed Electromagnetic Field (PEMF) Therapy is a non-invasive and safe form of therapy that uses low-frequency electromagnetic waves to stimulate the body's cells and promote healing. One of the most common uses of PEMF Therapy is for pain management. In this chapter, we will explore how PEMF Therapy can help with pain, types of pain that can be treated with PEMF Therapy, and research studies on PEMF Therapy and pain management.

How PEMF Therapy Can Help with Pain

PEMF Therapy can help with pain by reducing inflammation, improving circulation, and promoting cellular repair and regeneration. When applied to the affected area, PEMF Therapy increases the production of nitric oxide, a molecule that dilates blood vessels and improves blood flow. This increased blood flow can help reduce inflammation and swelling, which can alleviate pain. PEMF Therapy can also stimulate the production of endorphins, which are natural painkillers produced by the body.

Types of Pain that Can be Treated with PEMF Therapy

PEMF Therapy can be used to treat a variety of pain conditions, including:

- Arthritis
- Fibromyalgia
- Back pain
- Neck pain
- Joint pain
- Muscle pain

- Postoperative pain
- Neuropathic pain

Research Studies on PEMF Therapy and Pain Management

There is a growing body of research supporting the use of PEMF Therapy for pain management. A review of multiple studies on PEMF Therapy and pain management found that PEMF Therapy was effective in reducing pain in individuals with various pain conditions, including arthritis, fibromyalgia, and postoperative pain.

In a randomized, double-blind, placebo-controlled trial, PEMF Therapy was found to significantly reduce pain in individuals with knee osteoarthritis. Another study found that PEMF Therapy was effective in reducing pain and improving physical function in individuals with fibromyalgia.

A study on PEMF Therapy for chronic lower back pain found that participants who received PEMF Therapy had significantly lower pain scores and higher functional scores compared to those who received placebo treatment.

Overall, the research on PEMF Therapy and pain management is promising, and suggests that PEMF Therapy may be an effective non-invasive treatment for various types of pain.

Conclusion

PEMF Therapy is a safe and non-invasive form of therapy that can help with pain management. By reducing inflammation, improving circulation, and promoting cellular repair and regeneration, PEMF Therapy can help alleviate pain in individuals with various pain conditions, including arthritis, fibromyalgia, and back pain. Research studies have found PEMF Therapy to be effective in reducing pain and improving function in individuals with various types of pain. If you suffer from chronic pain, speak with your healthcare provider about whether PEMF Therapy may be a viable treatment option for you.

CHAPTER 5: Using PEMF Therapy for Improved Circulation

One of the benefits of PEMF Therapy is improved circulation. In this chapter, we will explore how PEMF Therapy can improve circulation, conditions that can benefit from improved circulation, and research studies on PEMF Therapy and improved circulation.

How PEMF Therapy Can Improve Circulation

PEMF Therapy can improve circulation by increasing the production of nitric oxide, a molecule that dilates blood vessels and improves blood flow. This increased blood flow can help deliver oxygen and nutrients to the body's tissues, which can promote healing and reduce inflammation. PEMF Therapy can also help stimulate the production of new blood vessels, a process known as angiogenesis, which can further improve circulation.

Conditions that Can Benefit from Improved Circulation

PEMF Therapy can benefit a variety of conditions that are related to poor circulation, including:

Peripheral artery disease
Diabetic neuropathy
Chronic wounds
Raynaud's disease
Migraines
In peripheral artery disease, the arteries that supply blood to the legs become narrowed, which can lead to poor circulation and pain. PEMF Therapy can help improve circulation in the legs, reducing pain and promoting healing.

Diabetic neuropathy is a complication of diabetes that can cause numbness, tingling, and pain in the feet and legs. Poor circulation is a common cause of diabetic neuropathy, and PEMF Therapy can help improve circulation and reduce the symptoms of diabetic neuropathy.

Chronic wounds, such as bedsores or diabetic foot ulcers, can be slow to heal due to poor circulation. PEMF Therapy can help improve circulation and promote the healing of chronic wounds.

Raynaud's disease is a condition in which the fingers and toes become cold and numb due to poor circulation. PEMF Therapy can help improve circulation in the affected areas, reducing the symptoms of Raynaud's disease.

Migraines are often associated with poor circulation, and PEMF Therapy can help improve blood flow to the brain, reducing the frequency and severity of migraines.

Research Studies on PEMF Therapy and Improved Circulation

There is a growing body of research supporting the use of PEMF Therapy for improved circulation. A randomized, double-blind, placebo-controlled trial found that PEMF Therapy was effective in improving circulation in individuals with peripheral artery disease.

A study on the use of PEMF Therapy for diabetic neuropathy found that participants who received PEMF Therapy had improved circulation in their feet and reduced symptoms compared to those who received sham treatment.

Another study found that PEMF Therapy was effective in promoting the healing of chronic wounds in individuals with diabetes.

Overall, the research on PEMF Therapy and improved circulation is promising, and suggests that PEMF Therapy may be an effective non-invasive treatment for a variety of conditions related to poor circulation.

CHAPTER 6: Using PEMF Therapy for Inflammation

One of the benefits of PEMF Therapy is reducing inflammation. In this chapter, we will explore how PEMF Therapy can reduce inflammation, conditions that can benefit from reduced inflammation, and research studies on PEMF Therapy and inflammation.

How PEMF Therapy Can Reduce Inflammation

PEMF Therapy can reduce inflammation by modulating the immune system and reducing the production of inflammatory cytokines. PEMF Therapy has been shown to reduce the expression of pro-inflammatory genes, such as TNF-alpha and IL-1 beta. This reduction in pro-inflammatory cytokines can lead to a decrease in inflammation and pain.

PEMF Therapy can also help increase circulation, which can aid in reducing inflammation. Increased circulation can help deliver oxygen and nutrients to the body's tissues, promoting healing and reducing inflammation.

Conditions that Can Benefit from Reduced Inflammation

PEMF Therapy can benefit a variety of conditions that are related to inflammation, including:

Arthritis
Fibromyalgia
Chronic pain
Chronic fatigue syndrome
Autoimmune diseases
Arthritis is a condition in which the joints become inflamed, causing pain and stiffness. PEMF Therapy can help reduce inflammation in the joints, decreasing pain and promoting healing.

Fibromyalgia is a chronic pain condition that is often associated with inflammation. PEMF Therapy can help reduce inflammation and pain in individuals with fibromyalgia.

Chronic pain is often related to inflammation. PEMF Therapy can help reduce inflammation, leading to a decrease in chronic pain.

Chronic fatigue syndrome is a condition that is associated with inflammation. PEMF Therapy can help reduce inflammation and improve energy levels in individuals with chronic fatigue syndrome.

Autoimmune diseases, such as rheumatoid arthritis and lupus, are caused by an overactive immune system that results in chronic inflammation. PEMF Therapy can help modulate the immune system and reduce the production of inflammatory cytokines, leading to a reduction in inflammation and an improvement in symptoms.

Research Studies on PEMF Therapy and Inflammation

There is a growing body of research supporting the use of PEMF Therapy for reducing inflammation. A study on the use of PEMF Therapy for knee osteoarthritis found that participants who received PEMF Therapy had a significant reduction in pain and inflammation compared to those who received sham treatment.

A randomized, double-blind, placebo-controlled trial found that PEMF Therapy was effective in reducing pain and inflammation in individuals with fibromyalgia.

Another study on the use of PEMF Therapy for chronic pain found that participants who received PEMF Therapy had a significant reduction in pain and inflammation compared to those who received sham treatment.

Overall, the research on PEMF Therapy and inflammation is promising, and suggests that PEMF Therapy may be an effective non-invasive treatment for a variety of conditions related to inflammation.

CHAPTER 7: Using PEMF Therapy for Healing and Recovery

One of the key benefits of PEMF Therapy is its ability to enhance healing and recovery. This can be particularly useful for individuals who have suffered injuries or undergone surgeries. PEMF Therapy can help accelerate the body's natural healing process by increasing blood flow, stimulating tissue growth, and reducing inflammation. This can help individuals recover more quickly and with fewer complications.

Conditions that can benefit from enhanced healing and recovery through PEMF Therapy include:

Arthritis and joint pain: PEMF Therapy has been shown to reduce joint pain and inflammation in individuals with arthritis. It can also improve joint flexibility and range of motion.

Bone fractures: PEMF Therapy has been shown to promote bone healing and reduce the time it takes for fractures to heal.

Post-operative recovery: PEMF Therapy can help reduce pain and inflammation following surgery and speed up the healing process.

Sports injuries: PEMF Therapy can be used to treat sports injuries, including sprains, strains, and muscle tears. It can help reduce pain and inflammation and speed up the healing process.

Chronic pain: PEMF Therapy has been shown to be effective in reducing chronic pain, including back pain and fibromyalgia.

There have been numerous research studies conducted on PEMF Therapy and its effects on healing and recovery. One study published in the Journal of Orthopaedic Surgery and Research found that PEMF Therapy was effective in reducing pain and improving mobility in individuals with knee osteoarthritis. Another study published in the Journal of International Medical Research found that PEMF Therapy was effective in reducing pain and improving function in individuals with chronic low back pain.

CHAPTER 8: <u>Using PEMF Therapy for Better Sleep</u>

One of the key benefits of PEMF Therapy is its ability to improve sleep quality. This can be particularly useful for individuals who struggle with insomnia, sleep apnea, or other sleep-related issues. PEMF Therapy has been shown to help regulate the body's natural sleep cycle, which can lead to better sleep and improved overall well-being.

Conditions that can benefit from improved sleep through PEMF Therapy include:

Insomnia: PEMF Therapy can help individuals fall asleep faster, stay asleep longer, and wake up feeling more rested.

Sleep apnea: PEMF Therapy can help improve the quality of sleep in individuals with sleep apnea, leading to reduced snoring, better breathing, and improved overall health.

Restless leg syndrome: PEMF Therapy can help reduce the symptoms of restless leg syndrome, such as leg twitching and discomfort, leading to better sleep.

Fibromyalgia: PEMF Therapy has been shown to improve sleep quality in individuals with fibromyalgia, reducing fatigue and improving overall well-being.

Chronic pain: PEMF Therapy can help reduce chronic pain, which can interfere with sleep, leading to better overall sleep quality.

There have been numerous research studies conducted on PEMF Therapy and its effects on sleep. One study published in the Journal of Sleep Research found that PEMF Therapy was effective in improving sleep quality in individuals with chronic pain. Another study published in the Journal of Alternative and Complementary Medicine found that PEMF Therapy was effective in improving sleep quality in individuals with fibromyalgia.

CHAPTER 9: Using PEMF Therapy for Stress and Anxiety

PEMF Therapy has been known to be a powerful tool in reducing stress and anxiety levels in the body. Stress and anxiety are common mental health issues that can significantly affect an individual's overall well-being. When the body is exposed to stress, it activates the sympathetic nervous system, leading to an increase in heart rate, blood pressure and cortisol levels. PEMF Therapy can help regulate the body's natural stress response, leading to reduced stress and anxiety levels and improved overall well-being.

Individuals who suffer from chronic stress, anxiety or other mood-related issues can benefit immensely from PEMF Therapy. By stimulating cellular regeneration and increasing circulation in the body, PEMF Therapy can help to reduce the symptoms of various conditions, including:

Generalized Anxiety Disorder: Generalized Anxiety Disorder (GAD) is a common condition that is characterized by excessive worry and restlessness. PEMF Therapy has been shown to help reduce the symptoms of GAD, leading to improved overall mental health.

Depression: Depression is a mood disorder that is characterized by feelings of sadness, low mood and lack of energy. PEMF Therapy has been shown to be effective in reducing the symptoms of depression, leading to improved overall mental health.

Post-Traumatic Stress Disorder (PTSD): Post-Traumatic Stress Disorder (PTSD) is a condition that is triggered by a traumatic event. Symptoms include flashbacks and anxiety. PEMF Therapy can help reduce the symptoms of PTSD, leading to improved overall well-being.

Chronic Pain: Chronic pain is a common condition that can cause significant stress and anxiety. PEMF Therapy can help reduce chronic pain, which can lead to reduced stress and anxiety levels.

Insomnia: Insomnia is a sleep disorder that can significantly affect an individual's overall well-being. PEMF Therapy can help improve sleep quality, which can lead to reduced stress and anxiety levels.

Research studies have been conducted to examine the effects of PEMF Therapy on stress and anxiety. One study published in the Journal of Affective Disorders found that PEMF Therapy was effective in reducing symptoms of anxiety and depression in individuals with bipolar disorder. Another study published in the Journal of Psychiatric Research found that PEMF Therapy was effective in reducing symptoms of anxiety in individuals with PTSD.

CHAPTER 10: Using PEMF Therapy for Athletic Performance

PEMF Therapy has become increasingly popular among athletes due to its ability to enhance athletic performance in several ways. Its ability to stimulate cellular regeneration and increase circulation in the body has been shown to improve athletic recovery, reduce pain and inflammation, and increase energy levels. In addition, it can improve sleep quality, reduce stress and anxiety, and enhance overall well-being, all of which can positively impact athletic performance.

PEMF Therapy is a highly versatile therapy that can benefit a wide range of athletes, including those who participate in high-intensity training, endurance sports, and competitive sports. Athletes who are prone to injuries, such as runners, football players, and basketball players, can benefit from PEMF Therapy as it helps to accelerate the healing process.

Numerous research studies have been conducted to investigate the effects of PEMF Therapy on athletic performance. A study published in the Journal of Sports Science and Medicine found that PEMF Therapy can improve muscle strength and flexibility in athletes. Similarly, a study published in the Journal of Athletic Training showed that PEMF Therapy can reduce muscle soreness and pain in athletes.

In a randomized, double-blind, placebo-controlled study on 21 elite male handball players, PEMF Therapy was found to be effective in reducing muscle fatigue, increasing muscular performance, and improving vertical jumping height. In another randomized, double-blind, placebo-controlled study on 30 healthy male volunteers, PEMF Therapy significantly increased peak power output and time to exhaustion during high-intensity exercise.

PEMF Therapy has also been found to be effective in improving muscle recovery and reducing muscle damage in long-distance runners. A study published in the Journal of Exercise Physiology found that PEMF Therapy can reduce muscle damage and improve muscle recovery in marathon runners. In addition, another study published in the Journal of Strength and Conditioning Research showed that PEMF Therapy can significantly improve muscle endurance and maximal oxygen uptake in soccer players.

In conclusion, PEMF Therapy has demonstrated significant potential in enhancing athletic performance. Its ability to stimulate cellular regeneration and increase circulation can help athletes recover faster from injuries, reduce pain and inflammation, and increase energy levels. Furthermore, it can improve sleep quality, reduce stress and anxiety, and enhance overall well-being, all of which can have a positive impact on athletic performance. The numerous research studies conducted have shown promising results, making PEMF Therapy a valuable tool for athletes looking to maximize their athletic potential.

CHAPTER 11: Using PEMF Therapy for Cognitive Function

PEMF therapy has been gaining popularity as an alternative treatment for a variety of health conditions, including those related to cognitive function. The therapy uses electromagnetic fields to stimulate cellular activity in the body, which can lead to improved cognitive function in individuals with certain conditions. In this article, we will explore how PEMF therapy can enhance cognitive function, which conditions can benefit from it, and the research studies that have been conducted on the therapy.

How PEMF Therapy can Enhance Cognitive Function:

Increased Blood Flow to the Brain: PEMF therapy has been shown to increase blood flow to the brain, which can lead to improved cognitive function. Studies have shown that increased blood flow to the brain can improve memory, attention, and information processing speed.

Improved Neuroplasticity: Neuroplasticity is the brain's ability to change and adapt in response to new experiences. PEMF therapy can enhance neuroplasticity by stimulating the growth of new neurons and synapses in the brain, which can lead to improved cognitive function.

Reduced Inflammation: Inflammation in the brain can lead to cognitive decline. PEMF therapy has been shown to reduce inflammation in the brain, which can help to improve cognitive function.

Enhanced Brain Connectivity: PEMF therapy can enhance connectivity between different regions of the brain, which can lead to improved cognitive function. Improved connectivity can lead to improved memory, attention, and cognitive flexibility.

Conditions that can Benefit from Enhanced Cognitive Function through PEMF Therapy:

Dementia: PEMF therapy has been shown to improve cognitive function in individuals with dementia. A study published in the Journal of Alzheimer's Disease found that PEMF therapy can improve cognitive function and quality of life in individuals with Alzheimer's disease.

Traumatic Brain Injury (TBI): TBI can lead to cognitive impairment. PEMF therapy has been shown to improve cognitive function in individuals with TBI. A study published in the Journal of Neurotrauma found that PEMF therapy can improve cognitive function in individuals with mild TBI.

Depression: Depression can lead to cognitive impairment. PEMF therapy has been shown to improve cognitive function in individuals with depression. A study published in the Journal of Affective Disorders found that PEMF therapy can improve cognitive function in individuals with depression.

Research Studies on PEMF Therapy and Cognitive Function:

A study published in the Journal of Alzheimer's Disease found that PEMF therapy can improve cognitive function and quality of life in individuals with Alzheimer's disease.

A study published in the Journal of Neurotrauma found that PEMF therapy can improve cognitive function in individuals with mild TBI.

A study published in the Journal of Affective Disorders found that PEMF therapy can improve cognitive function in individuals with depression.

A study published in the Journal of Translational Medicine found that PEMF therapy can improve cognitive function and quality of life in individuals with multiple sclerosis.

A study published in the Journal of Neural Regeneration Research found that PEMF therapy can improve cognitive function in individuals with Parkinson's disease.

In conclusion, PEMF therapy has been shown to enhance cognitive function by increasing blood flow to the brain, improving neuroplasticity, reducing inflammation, and enhancing brain connectivity. The therapy can benefit individuals with conditions such as dementia, TBI, and depression. Research studies have shown that PEMF therapy can improve cognitive function in individuals with these conditions. If you are considering PEMF therapy for cognitive function, it is important to consult with a healthcare professional to determine if it is right for you.

CHAPTER 12: Choosing the Right PEMF Device

PEMF therapy has been shown to provide a number of health benefits, including improved sleep, reduced pain and inflammation, enhanced athletic performance, and reduced stress and anxiety. As a result, more and more people are looking to purchase PEMF devices for home use. However, with so many different PEMF devices on the market, it can be difficult to know which one to choose. In this article, we'll explore the factors you should consider when choosing a PEMF device, take a look at some popular devices on the market, and provide tips for making a smart purchase.

Factors to consider when choosing a PEMF device:

Intended Use: The first factor to consider when choosing a PEMF device is what you want to use it for. Different PEMF devices may be designed for specific purposes, such as treating pain, improving sleep, or enhancing athletic performance. Make sure you choose a device that is designed for your specific needs.

Frequency and Intensity: The frequency and intensity of the electromagnetic waves generated by a PEMF device are important factors to consider. Higher frequencies and intensities may be more effective for treating certain conditions, but they may also have more potential side effects. Make sure to choose a device with the appropriate frequency and intensity for your needs.

Waveform: The waveform of the electromagnetic waves generated by a PEMF device can also affect its effectiveness. Some devices use a sawtooth waveform, while others use a sine wave or a square wave. Each waveform has its own unique properties, so make sure to choose a device with the appropriate waveform for your needs.

Portability: Some PEMF devices are portable and can be used on the go, while others are designed for use in a specific location, such as a home or office. If you plan to use your device while traveling or on the go, make sure to choose a portable device that is easy to transport.

Cost: PEMF devices can range in price from a few hundred dollars to several thousand dollars. Make sure to choose a device that fits your budget and provides good value for the price.

<u>**Popular PEMF devices on the market:**</u>

EarthPulse: EarthPulse is a popular PEMF device that is designed to improve sleep, increase energy, and reduce pain and inflammation. It uses a sine wave at a frequency of 9.6 Hz and has a portable design.

Pulse Centers XL Pro: The Pulse Centers XL Pro is a high-end PEMF device designed for use in a clinical setting. It offers a range of waveforms and frequencies, and can be used to treat a variety of conditions, including pain, inflammation, and anxiety.

OMI PEMF Therapy Mat: The OMI PEMF Therapy Mat is a portable mat that uses a square wave at a frequency of 8 Hz. It is designed to improve circulation, reduce pain and inflammation, and enhance athletic performance.

<u>**Tips for purchasing a PEMF device:**</u>

Do Your Research: Before purchasing a PEMF device, make sure to do your research. Look for reviews from other users, and make sure to choose a device from a reputable manufacturer.

Consult with a Professional: If you are unsure which PEMF device is right for your needs, consider consulting with a healthcare professional or a PEMF therapy practitioner.

Consider the Warranty: Make sure to choose a device with a good warranty that covers any potential defects or malfunctions.

Try Before You Buy: If possible, try out a PEMF device before you buy it. Many practitioners and clinics offer trial sessions that allow you to experience the benefits of PEMF therapy firsthand.

In conclusion, choosing the right PEMF device requires careful consideration of factors such as intended use, frequency and intensity, waveform, portability, and cost

CHAPTER 13: How to Use PEMF Therapy

How to Prepare for a PEMF Therapy Session:

Before undergoing a PEMF therapy session, there are a few steps you can take to ensure that you get the most out of the experience. Here are some tips to help you prepare:

Dress Comfortably: Wear loose-fitting, comfortable clothing that will not interfere with the therapy session.

Stay Hydrated: Drink plenty of water before and after your session to help your body flush out toxins and enhance the therapy's effects.

Remove Metal Objects: Remove any metal jewelry or objects, as they can interfere with the electromagnetic field.

Relax: Try to relax and clear your mind before the session to help you get the full benefits of the therapy.

How to Use a PEMF Device at Home:

PEMF devices are available for home use, making it convenient for individuals to use them whenever they need to. Here are some steps to follow when using a PEMF device at home:

Read the Instructions: Make sure to read and follow the manufacturer's instructions carefully before using the device.

Choose the Right Frequency: Different frequencies may be used for different conditions, so choose the appropriate frequency for the desired result.

Positioning: Position the device correctly and securely on the area that needs treatment, and use the appropriate intensity level.

Duration: Follow the recommended time for each session and do not exceed it.

Regular Use: To achieve the best results, use the PEMF device regularly and consistently over time.

Tips for Maximizing the Benefits of PEMF Therapy:

To maximize the benefits of PEMF therapy, there are a few things you can do:

Combine with Other Therapies: PEMF therapy can be used in combination with other therapies, such as physical therapy, chiropractic care, or massage, to enhance its effects.

Consult with a Professional: It is recommended to consult with a qualified healthcare professional before using PEMF therapy to ensure that it is appropriate for your specific needs and medical conditions.

Be Consistent: Use PEMF therapy regularly and consistently over time to achieve the best results.

Adjust Frequency and Intensity: Adjust the frequency and intensity level of the device as needed for different conditions or stages of recovery.

Stay Active: Combining PEMF therapy with regular exercise and a healthy lifestyle can help to optimize its effects.

In conclusion, PEMF therapy can be a powerful tool for improving health and wellness. By following the tips and guidelines above, individuals can prepare for a session, use a PEMF device at home, and maximize its benefits. However, it is important to consult with a qualified healthcare professional before using PEMF therapy, especially if you have a medical condition or are taking any medication. With the right approach, PEMF therapy can be a safe and effective way to support overall health and well-being.